AIR FRYER RECIPES

MOUTH-WATERING RECIPES

JAMES WILLIAMS

Table of Contents

Introduction

Are you always looking for easier and more modern ways to cook the best meals for you and all your loved ones?

Are you constantly searching for useful kitchen appliances that will make your work in the kitchen more fun?

Well, you don't need to search anymore! We present to you today the best kitchen appliance available these days on the market: the air fryer!

Air fryers are simply the best kitchen tools for so many reasons. Are you interested in discovering more about air fryers? Then, pay attention next!

First of all, you need to know that air fryers are special and revolutionary kitchen appliances that cook your food using the circulation of hot air. These tools use a special technology called rapid air technology. Therefore, all the food you cook in these fryers is succulent on the inside and perfectly cooked on the outside.

The next thing you need to find out about air fryers is that they allow you to cook, bake, steam and roast pretty much everything you can imagine.

Last but not least, you should know that air fryers help you cook your meals in a much healthier way.
So many people all over the world just fell in love with this great and amazing tool and now it's your turn to become one of them.

So...long story short, we recommend you to purchase an air fryer right away and to get your hands on this cooking journal as soon as possible!

We can assure you that all the meals you cook in your air fryer will taste so good and that everyone will admire your cooking skills from now one!

So, let's get started!
Have fun cooking with your great air fryer!

Air Fryer Lunch Recipes

Lentils Fritters

Preparation time: 10 minutes **Cooking time:** 10 minutes
Servings: 2

Ingredients:

- 1 cup yellow lentils, soaked in water for 1 hour and drained
- 1 hot chili pepper, chopped
- 1 inch ginger piece, grated
- ½ teaspoon turmeric powder
- 1 teaspoon garam masala
- 1 teaspoon baking powder
- Salt and black pepper to the taste
- 2 teaspoons olive oil
- 1/3 cup water
- ½ cup cilantro, chopped
- 1 and ½ cup spinach, chopped
- 4 garlic cloves, minced
- ¾ cup red onion, chopped
- Mint chutney for serving

Directions:

1. In your blender, mix lentils with chili pepper, ginger, turmeric, garam masala, baking powder, salt, pepper, olive oil, water, cilantro, spinach, onion and garlic, blend well and shape medium balls out of this mix.
2. Place them all in your preheated air fryer at 400 degrees F and cook for 10 minutes.
3. Serve your veggie fritters with a side salad for lunch.

Enjoy!

Nutrition: calories 142, fat 2, fiber 8, carbs 12, protein 4

Lunch Potato Salad

Preparation time: 10 minutes **Cooking time:** 25 minutes

Servings: 4

Ingredients:

- 2 pound red potatoes, halved
- 2 tablespoons olive oil
- Salt and black pepper to the taste
- 2 green onions, chopped
- 1 red bell pepper, chopped
- 1/3 cup lemon juice
- 3 tablespoons mustard

Directions:

1. On your air fryer's basket, mix potatoes with half of the olive oil, salt and pepper and cook at 350 degrees F for 25 minutes shaking the fryer once.
2. In a bowl, mix onions with bell pepper and roasted potatoes and toss.

3. In a small bowl, mix lemon juice with the rest of the oil and mustard and whisk really well.
4. Add this to potato salad, toss well and serve for lunch.

Enjoy!

Nutrition: calories 211, fat 6, fiber 8, carbs 12, protein 4

Corn Casserole

Preparation time: 10 minutes **Cooking time:** 15 minutes
Servings: 4

Ingredients:

- 2 cups corn
- 3 tablespoons flour
- 1 egg
- ¼ cup milk
- ½ cup light cream
- ½ cup Swiss cheese, grated
- 2 tablespoons butter
- Salt and black pepper to the taste
- Cooking spray

Directions:

1. In a bowl, mix corn with flour, egg, milk, light cream, cheese, salt, pepper and butter and stir well.
2. Grease your air fryer's pan with cooking spray, pour cream mix, spread and cook at 320 degrees F for 15 minutes.
3. Serve warm for lunch.

Enjoy!

Nutrition: calories 281, fat 7, fiber 8, carbs 9, protein 6

Bacon and Garlic Pizzas

Preparation time: 10 minutes **Cooking time:** 10 minutes
Servings: 4

Ingredients:

- 4 dinner rolls, frozen
- 4 garlic cloves minced
- ½ teaspoon oregano dried
- ½ teaspoon garlic powder
- 1 cup tomato sauce
- 8 bacon slices, cooked and chopped
- 1 and ¼ cups cheddar cheese, grated
- Cooking spray

Directions:

1. Place dinner rolls on a working surface and press them to obtain 4 ovals.
2. Spray each oval with cooking spray, transfer them to your air fryer and cook them at 370 degrees F for 2 minutes.

3. Spread tomato sauce on each oval, divide garlic, sprinkle oregano and garlic powder and top with bacon and cheese.
4. Return pizzas to your heated air fryer and cook them at 370 degrees F for 8 minutes more.
5. Serve them warm for lunch.

Enjoy!

Nutrition: calories 217, fat 5, fiber 8, carbs 12, protein 4

Sweet and Sour Sausage Mix

Preparation time: 10 minutes **Cooking time:** 10 minutes

Servings: 4

Ingredients:

- 1 pound sausages, sliced
- 1 red bell pepper, cut into strips
- ½ cup yellow onion, chopped
- 3 tablespoons brown sugar
- 1/3 cup ketchup
- 2 tablespoons mustard
- 2 tablespoons apple cider vinegar
- ½ cup chicken stock

Directions:

1. In a bowl, mix sugar with ketchup, mustard, stock and vinegar and whisk well.
2. In your air fryer's pan, mix sausage slices with bell pepper, onion and sweet and sour mix, toss and cook at 350 degrees F for 10 minutes.
3. Divide into bowls and serve for lunch.

Enjoy!

Nutrition: calories 162, fat 6, fiber 9, carbs 12, protein 6

Meatballs and Tomato Sauce

Preparation time: 10 minutes **Cooking time:** 15 minutes

Servings: 4

Ingredients:

- 1 pound lean beef, ground
- 3 green onions, chopped
- 2 garlic cloves, minced
- 1 egg yolk
- ¼ cup bread crumbs
- Salt and black pepper to the taste
- 1 tablespoon olive oil
- 16 ounces tomato sauce
- 2 tablespoons mustard

Directions:

1. In a bowl, mix beef with onion, garlic, egg yolk, bread crumbs, salt and pepper, stir well and shape medium meatballs out of this mix.
2. Grease meatballs with the oil, place them in your air fryer and cook them at 400 degrees F for 10 minutes.

3. In a bowl, mix tomato sauce with mustard, whisk, add over meatballs, toss them and cook at 400 degrees F for 5 minutes more.
4. Divide meatballs and sauce on plates and serve for lunch.

Enjoy!

Nutrition: calories 300, fat 8, fiber 9, carbs 16, protein 5

Stuffed Meatballs

Preparation time: 10 minutes **Cooking time:** 10 minutes
Servings: 4

Ingredients:

- 1/3 cup bread crumbs
- 3 tablespoons milk
- 1 tablespoon ketchup
- 1 egg
- ½ teaspoon marjoram, dried
- Salt and black pepper to the taste
- 1 pound lean beef, ground
- 20 cheddar cheese cubes
- 1 tablespoon olive oil

Directions:

1. In a bowl, mix bread crumbs with ketchup, milk, marjoram, salt, pepper and egg and whisk well.
2. Add beef, stir and shape 20 meatballs out of this mix.
3. Shape each meatball around a cheese cube, drizzle the oil over them and rub.
4. Place all meatballs in your preheated air fryer and cook at 390 degrees F for 10 minutes.
5. Serve them for lunch with a side salad.

Enjoy!

Nutrition: calories 200, fat 5, fiber 8, carbs 12, protein 5

Steaks and Cabbage

Preparation time: 10 minutes **Cooking time:** 10 minutes
Servings: 4

Ingredients:

- ½ pound sirloin steak, cut into strips
- 2 teaspoons cornstarch
- 1 tablespoon peanut oil
- 2 cups green cabbage, chopped
- 1 yellow bell pepper, chopped
- 2 green onions, chopped
- 2 garlic cloves, minced
- Salt and black pepper to the taste

Directions:

1. In a bowl, mix cabbage with salt, pepper and peanut oil, toss, transfer to air fryer's basket, cook at 370 degrees F for 4 minutes and transfer to a bowl.
2. Add steak strips to your air fryer, also add green onions, bell pepper, garlic, salt and pepper, toss and cook for 5 minutes.
3. Add over cabbage, toss, divide among plates and serve for lunch.

Enjoy!

Nutrition: calories 282, fat 6, fiber 8, carbs 14, protein 6

Succulent Lunch Turkey Breast

Preparation time: 10 minutes **Cooking time:** 47 minutes

Servings: 4

Ingredients:

- 1 big turkey breast
- 2 teaspoons olive oil
- ½ teaspoon smoked paprika
- 1 teaspoon thyme, dried
- ½ teaspoon sage, dried
- Salt and black pepper to the taste
- 2 tablespoons mustard
- ¼ cup maple syrup
- 1 tablespoon butter, soft

Directions:

1. Brush turkey breast with the olive oil, season with salt, pepper, thyme, paprika and sage, rub, place in your air fryer's basket and fry at 350 degrees F for 25 minutes.
2. Flip turkey, cook for 10 minutes more, flip one more time and cook for another 10 minutes.

3. Meanwhile, heat up a pan with the butter over medium heat, add mustard and maple syrup, stir well, cook for a couple of minutes and take off heat.
4. Slice turkey breast, divide among plates and serve with the maple glaze drizzled on top.

Enjoy!

Nutrition: calories 280, fat 2, fiber 7, carbs 16, protein 14

Italian Eggplant Sandwich

Preparation time: 10 minutes **Cooking time:** 16 minutes
Servings: 2

Ingredients:

- 1 eggplant, sliced
- 2 teaspoons parsley, dried
- Salt and black pepper to the taste
- ½ cup breadcrumbs
- ½ teaspoon Italian seasoning
- ½ teaspoon garlic powder
- ½ teaspoon onion powder
- 2 tablespoons milk
- 4 bread slices
- Cooking spray
- ½ cup mayonnaise
- ¾ cup tomato sauce
- 2 cups mozzarella cheese, grated

Directions:

1. Season eggplant slices with salt and pepper, leave aside for 10 minutes and then pat dry them well.

2. In a bowl, mix parsley with breadcrumbs, Italian seasoning, onion and garlic powder, salt and black pepper and stir.
3. In another bowl, mix milk with mayo and whisk well.
4. Brush eggplant slices with mayo mix, dip them in breadcrumbs, place them in your air fryer's basket, spray with cooking oil and cook them at 400 degrees F for 15 minutes, flipping them after 8 minutes.
5. Brush each bread slice with olive oil and arrange 2 on a working surface.
6. Add mozzarella and parmesan on each, add baked eggplant slices, spread tomato sauce and basil and top with the other bread slices, greased side down.
7. Divide sandwiches on plates, cut them in halves and serve for lunch.

Enjoy!

Nutrition: calories 324, fat 16, fiber 4, carbs 39, protein 12

Creamy Chicken Stew

Preparation time: 10 minutes **Cooking time:** 25 minutes
Servings: 4

Ingredients:

- 1 and ½ cups canned cream of celery soup
- 6 chicken tenders
- Salt and black pepper to the taste
- 2 potatoes, chopped
- 1 bay leaf
- 1 thyme spring, chopped
- 1 tablespoon milk
- 1 egg yolk
- ½ cup heavy cream

Directions:

1. In a bowl, mix chicken with cream of celery, potatoes, heavy cream, bay leaf, thyme, salt and pepper, toss, pour into your air fryer's pan and cook at 320 degrees F for 25 minutes.
2. Leave your stew to cool down a bit, discard bay leaf, divide among plates and serve right away.

Enjoy!

Nutrition: calories 300, fat 11, fiber 2, carbs 23, protein 14

Lunch Pork and Potatoes

Preparation time: 10 minutes **Cooking time:** 25 minutes

Servings: 2

Ingredients:

- 2 pounds pork loin
- Salt and black pepper to the taste
- 2 red potatoes, cut into medium wedges
- ½ teaspoon garlic powder
- ½ teaspoon red pepper flakes
- 1 teaspoon parsley, dried
- A drizzle of balsamic vinegar

Directions:

1. In your air fryer's pan, mix pork with potatoes, salt, pepper, garlic powder, pepper flakes, parsley and vinegar, toss and cook at 390 degrees F for 25 minutes.
2. Slice pork, divide it and potatoes on plates and serve for lunch.

Enjoy!

Nutrition: calories 400, fat 15, fiber 7, carbs 27, protein 20

Turkey Cakes

Preparation time: 10 minutes **Cooking time:** 10 minutes
Servings: 4

Ingredients:

- 6 mushrooms, chopped
- 1 teaspoon garlic powder
- 1 teaspoon onion powder
- Salt and black pepper to the taste
- 1 and ¼ pounds turkey meat, ground
- Cooking spray
- Tomato sauce for serving

Directions:

1. In your blender, mix mushrooms with salt and pepper, pulse well and transfer to a bowl.
2. Add turkey, onion powder, garlic powder, salt and pepper, stir and shape cakes out of this mix.
3. Spray them with cooking spray, transfer them to your air fryer and cook at 320 degrees F for 10 minutes.
4. Serve them with tomato sauce on the side and a tasty side salad.

Enjoy!

Nutrition: calories 202, fat 6, fiber 3, carbs 17, protein 10

Cheese Ravioli and Marinara Sauce

Preparation time: 10 minutes **Cooking time:** 8 minutes

Servings: 6

Ingredients:

- 20 ounces cheese ravioli
- 10 ounces marinara sauce
- 1 tablespoon olive oil
- 1 cup buttermilk
- 2 cups bread crumbs
- ¼ cup parmesan, grated

Directions:

1. Put buttermilk in a bowl and breadcrumbs in another bowl.
2. Dip ravioli in buttermilk, then in breadcrumbs and place them in your air fryer on a baking sheet.
3. Drizzle olive oil over them, cook at 400 degrees F for 5 minutes, divide them on plates, sprinkle parmesan on top and serve for lunch

Enjoy!

Nutrition: calories 270, fat 12, fiber 6, carbs 30, protein 15

Beef Stew

Preparation time: 10 minutes **Cooking time:** 20 minutes
Servings: 4

Ingredients:

- 2 pounds beef meat, cut into medium chunks
- 2 carrots, chopped
- 4 potatoes, chopped
- Salt and black pepper to the taste
- 1 quart veggie stock
- ½ teaspoon smoked paprika
- A handful thyme, chopped

Directions:

1. In a dish that fits your air fryer, mix beef with carrots, potatoes, stock, salt, pepper, paprika and thyme, stir, place in air fryer's basket and cook at 375 degrees F for 20 minutes.

2. Divide into bowls and serve right away for lunch.

Enjoy!

Nutrition: calories 260, fat 5, fiber 8, carbs 20, protein 22

Meatballs Sandwich

Preparation time: 10 minutes **Cooking time:** 22 minutes

Servings: 4

Ingredients:

- 3 baguettes, sliced more than halfway through
- 14 ounces beef, ground
- 7 ounces tomato sauce
- 1 small onion, chopped
- 1 egg, whisked
- 1 tablespoon bread crumbs
- 2 tablespoons cheddar cheese, grated
- 1 tablespoon oregano, chopped
- 1 tablespoon olive oil
- Salt and black pepper to the taste
- 1 teaspoon thyme, dried
- 1 teaspoon basil, dried

Directions:

1. In a bowl, combine meat with salt, pepper, onion, breadcrumbs, egg, cheese, oregano, thyme and basil,

stir, shape medium meatballs and add them to your air fryer after you've greased it with the oil.

2. Cook them at 375 degrees F for 12 minutes, flipping them halfway.
3. Add tomato sauce, cook meatballs for 10 minutes more and arrange them on sliced baguettes.
4. Serve them right away.

Enjoy!

Nutrition: calories 380, fat 5, fiber 6, carbs 34, protein 20

Bacon Pudding

Preparation time: 10 minutes **Cooking time:** 30 minutes
Servings: 6

Ingredients:

- 4 bacon strips, cooked and chopped
- 1 tablespoon butter, soft
- 2 cups corn
- 1 yellow onion, chopped
- ¼ cup celery, chopped
- ½ cup red bell pepper, chopped
- 1 teaspoon thyme, chopped
- 2 teaspoons garlic, minced
- Salt and black pepper to the taste
- ½ cup heavy cream
- 1 and ½ cups milk
- 3 eggs, whisked
- 3 cups bread, cubed
- 4 tablespoons parmesan, grated
- Cooking spray

Directions:

1. Grease your air fryer's pan with coking spray.
2. In a bowl, mix bacon with butter, corn, onion, bell pepper, celery, thyme, garlic, salt, pepper, milk, heavy cream, eggs and bread cubes, toss, pour into greased pan and sprinkle cheese all over
3. Add this to your preheated air fryer at 320 degrees and cook for 30 minutes.
4. Divide among plates and serve warm for a quick lunch.

Enjoy!

Nutrition: calories 276, fat 10, fiber 2, carbs 20, protein 10

Special Lunch Seafood Stew

Preparation time: 10 minutes **Cooking time:** 20 minutes
Servings: 4

Ingredients:

- 5 ounces white rice
- 2 ounces peas
- 1 red bell pepper, chopped
- 14 ounces white wine
- 3 ounces water
- 2 ounces squid pieces
- 7 ounces mussels
- 3 ounces sea bass fillet, skinless, boneless and chopped
- 6 scallops
- 3.5 ounces clams
- 4 shrimp
- 4 crayfish
- Salt and black pepper to the taste
- 1 tablespoon olive oil

Directions:

1. In your air fryer's pan, mix sea bass with shrimp, mussels, scallops, crayfish, clams and squid.
2. Add the oil, salt and pepper and toss to coat.
3. In a bowl, mix peas salt, pepper, bell pepper and rice and stir.
4. Add this over seafood, also add whine and water, place pan in your air fryer and cook at 400 degrees F for 20 minutes, stirring halfway.
5. Divide into bowls and serve for lunch.

Enjoy!

Nutrition: calories 300, fat 12, fiber 2, carbs 23, protein 25

Air Fried Thai Salad

Preparation time: 10 minutes **Cooking time:** 5 minutes
Servings: 4

Ingredients:

- 1 cup carrots, grated
- 1 cup red cabbage, shredded
- A pinch of salt and black pepper
- A handful cilantro, chopped
- 1 small cucumber, chopped
- Juice from 1 lime
- 2 teaspoons red curry paste
- 12 big shrimp, cooked, peeled and deveined

Directions:

1. In a pan that fits your, mix cabbage with carrots, cucumber and shrimp, toss, introduce in your air fryer and cook at 360 degrees F for 5 minutes.
2. Add salt, pepper, cilantro, lime juice and red curry paste, toss again, divide among plates and serve right away.

Enjoy!

Nutrition: calories 172, fat 5, fiber 7, carbs 8, protein 5

Sweet Potato Lunch Casserole

Preparation time: 10 minutes **Cooking time:** 50 minutes
Servings: 6

Ingredients:

- 3 big sweet potatoes, pricked with a fork
- 1 cup chicken stock
- Salt and black pepper to the taste
- A pinch of cayenne pepper
- ¼ teaspoon nutmeg, ground
- 1/3 cup coconut cream

Directions:

1. Place sweet potatoes in your air fryer, cook them at 350 degrees F for 40 minutes, cool them down, peel, roughly chop and transfer to a pan that fits your air fryer.
2. Add stock, salt, pepper, cayenne and coconut cream, toss, introduce in your air fryer and cook at 360 degrees F for 10 minutes more.
3. Divide casserole into bowls and serve.

Enjoy!

Nutrition: calories 245, fat 4, fiber 5, carbs 10, protein 6

Zucchini Casserole

Preparation time: 10 minutes **Cooking time:** 16 minutes
Servings: 8

Ingredients:

- 1 cup veggie stock
- 2 tablespoons olive oil
- 2 sweet potatoes, peeled and cut into medium wedges
- 8 zucchinis, cut into medium wedges
- 2 yellow onions, chopped
- 1 cup coconut milk
- Salt and black pepper to the taste
- 1 tablespoon soy sauce
- ¼ teaspoon thyme, dried
- ¼ teaspoon rosemary, dried
- 4 tablespoons dill, chopped
- ½ teaspoon basil, chopped

Directions:

1. Heat up a pan that fits your air fryer with the oil over medium heat, add onion, stir and cook for 2 minutes.

2. Add zucchinis, thyme, rosemary, basil, potato, salt, pepper, stock, milk, soy sauce and dill, stir, introduce in your air fryer, cook at 360 degrees F for 14 minutes, divide among plates and serve right away.

Enjoy!

Nutrition: calories 133, fat 3, fiber 4, carbs 10, protein 5

Coconut and Chicken Casserole

Preparation time: 10 minutes **Cooking time:** 25 minutes

Servings: 4

Ingredients:

- 4 lime leaves, torn
- 1 cup veggie stock
- 1 lemongrass stalk, chopped
- 1 inch piece, grated
- 1 pound chicken breast, skinless, boneless and cut into thin strips
- 8 ounces mushrooms, chopped
- 4 Thai chilies, chopped
- 4 tablespoons fish sauce
- 6 ounces coconut milk
- ¼ cup lime juice
- ¼ cup cilantro, chopped
- Salt and black pepper to the taste

Directions:

1. Put stock into a pan that fits your air fryer, bring to a simmer over medium heat, add lemongrass, ginger and lime leaves, stir and cook for 10 minutes.
2. Strain soup, return to pan, add chicken, mushrooms, milk, chilies, fish sauce, lime juice, cilantro, salt and pepper, stir, introduce in your air fryer and cook at 360 degrees F for 15 minutes.
3. Divide into bowls and serve.

Enjoy!

Nutrition: calories 150, fat 4, fiber 4, carbs 6, protein 7

Turkey Burgers

Preparation time: 10 minutes **Cooking time:** 8 minutes
Servings: 4

Ingredients:

- 1 pound turkey meat, ground
- 1 shallot, minced
- A drizzle of olive oil
- 1 small jalapeno pepper, minced
- 2 teaspoons lime juice
- Zest from 1 lime, grated
- Salt and black pepper to the taste
- 1 teaspoon cumin, ground
- 1 teaspoon sweet paprika
- Guacamole for serving

Directions:

1. In a bowl, mix turkey meat with salt, pepper, cumin, paprika, shallot, jalapeno, lime juice and zest, stir well, shape burgers from this mix, drizzle the oil over them, introduce in preheated air fryer and cook them at 370 degrees F for 8 minutes on each side.
2. Divide among plates and serve with guacamole on top.

Enjoy!

Nutrition: calories 200, fat 12, fiber 0, carbs 0, protein 12

Salmon and Asparagus

Preparation time: 10 minutes **Cooking time:** 23 minutes

Servings: 4

Ingredients:

- 1 pound asparagus, trimmed
- 1 tablespoon olive oil
- A pinch of sweet paprika
- Salt and black pepper to the taste
- A pinch of garlic powder
- A pinch of cayenne pepper
- 1 red bell pepper, cut into halves
- 4 ounces smoked salmon

Directions:

1. Put asparagus spears and bell pepper on a lined baking sheet that fits your air fryer, add salt, pepper, garlic powder, paprika, olive oil, cayenne pepper, toss to coat, introduce in the fryer, cook at 390 degrees F for 8 minutes, flip and cook for 8 minutes more.
2. Add salmon, cook for 5 minutes, more, divide everything on plates and serve.

Enjoy!

Nutrition: calories 90, fat 1, fiber 1, carbs 1.2, protein 4

Easy Chicken Lunch

Preparation time: 10 minutes **Cooking time:** 20 minutes
Servings: 6

Ingredients:

- 1 bunch kale, chopped
- Salt and black pepper to the taste
- ¼ cup chicken stock
- 1 cup chicken, shredded
- 3 carrots, chopped
- 1 cup shiitake mushrooms, roughly sliced

Directions:

1. In a blender, mix stock with kale, pulse a few times and pour into a pan that fits your air fryer.
2. Add chicken, mushrooms, carrots, salt and pepper to the taste, toss, introduce in your air fryer and cook at 350 degrees F for 18 minutes.

Enjoy!

Nutrition: calories 180, fat 7, fiber 2, carbs 10, protein 5

Chicken and Corn Casserole

Preparation time: 10 minutes **Cooking time:** 30 minutes
Servings: 6

Ingredients:

- 1 cup clean chicken stock
- 2 teaspoons garlic powder
- Salt and black pepper to the taste
- 6 ounces canned coconut milk
- 1 and ½ cups green lentils
- 2 pounds chicken breasts, skinless, boneless and cubed
- 1/3 cup cilantro, chopped
- 3 cups corn
- 3 handfuls spinach
- 3 green onions, chopped

Directions:

1. In a pan that fits your air fryer, mix stock with coconut
   milk, salt, pepper, garlic powder, chicken and lentils.

2. Add corn, green onions, cilantro and spinach, stir well, introduce in your air fryer and cook at 350 degrees F for 30 minutes.

Enjoy!

Nutrition: calories 345, fat 12, fiber 10, carbs 20, protein 44

Chicken and Zucchini Lunch Mix

Preparation time: 10 minutes **Cooking time:** 20 minutes
Servings: 4

Ingredients:

- 4 zucchinis, cut with a spiralizer
- 1 pound chicken breasts, skinless, boneless and cubed
- 2 garlic cloves, minced
- 1 teaspoon olive oil
- Salt and black pepper to the taste
- 2 cups cherry tomatoes, halved
- ½ cup almonds, chopped

For the pesto:

- 2 cups basil
- 2 cups kale, chopped
- 1 tablespoon lemon juice
- 1 garlic clove
- ¾ cup pine nuts
- ½ cup olive oil
- A pinch of salt

Directions:

1. In your food processor, mix basil with kale, lemon juice, garlic, pine nuts, oil and a pinch of salt, pulse really well and leave aside.
2. Heat up a pan that fits your air fryer with the oil over medium heat, add garlic, stir and cook for 1 minute.
3. Add chicken, salt, pepper, stir, almonds, zucchini noodles, garlic, cherry tomatoes and the pesto you've made at the beginning, stir gently, introduce in preheated air fryer and cook at 360 degrees F for 17 minutes.
4. Divide among plates and serve for lunch.

Enjoy!

Nutrition: calories 344, fat 8, fiber 7, carbs 12, protein 16

Chicken, Beans, Corn and Quinoa Casserole

Preparation time: 10 minutes **Cooking time:** 30 minutes
Servings: 8

Ingredients:

- 1 cup quinoa, already cooked
- 3 cups chicken breast, cooked and shredded
- 14 ounces canned black beans
- 12 ounces corn
- ½ cup cilantro, chopped
- 6 kale leaves, chopped
- ½ cup green onions, chopped
- 1 cup clean tomato sauce
- 1 cup clean salsa
- 2 teaspoons chili powder
- 2 teaspoons cumin, ground
- 3 cups mozzarella cheese, shredded
- 1 tablespoon garlic powder
- Cooking spray
- 2 jalapeno peppers, chopped

Directions:

1. Spray a baking dish that fits your air fryer with cooking spray, add quinoa, chicken, black beans, corn, cilantro, kale, green onions, tomato sauce, salsa, chili powder, cumin, garlic powder, jalapenos and mozzarella, toss, introduce in your fryer and cook at 350 degrees F for 17 minutes.
2. Slice and serve warm for lunch.

Enjoy!

Nutrition: calories 365, fat 12, fiber 6, carbs 22, protein 26

Air Fryer Side Dish Recipes

Potato Wedges

Preparation time: 10 minutes **Cooking time:** 25 minutes
Servings: 4

Ingredients:

- 2 potatoes, cut into wedges
- 1 tablespoon olive oil
- Salt and black pepper to the taste
- 3 tablespoons sour cream
- 2 tablespoons sweet chili sauce

Directions:

1. In a bowl, mix potato wedges with oil, salt and pepper, toss well, add to air fryer's basket and cook at 360 degrees F for 25 minutes, flipping them once.
2. Divide potato wedges on plates, drizzle sour cream and chili sauce all over and serve them as a side dish.

Enjoy!

Nutrition: calories 171, fat 8, fiber 9, carbs 18, protein 7

Mushroom Side Dish

Preparation time: 10 minutes **Cooking time:** 8 minutes
Servings: 4

Ingredients:

- 10 button mushrooms, stems removed
- 1 tablespoon Italian seasoning
- Salt and black pepper to the taste
- 2 tablespoons cheddar cheese, grated
- 1 tablespoon olive oil
- 2 tablespoons mozzarella, grated
- 1 tablespoon dill, chopped

Directions:

1. In a bowl, mix mushrooms with Italian seasoning, salt, pepper, oil and dill and rub well.
2. Arrange mushrooms in your air fryer's basket, sprinkle mozzarella and cheddar in each and cook them at 360 degrees F for 8 minutes.
3. Divide them on plates and serve them as a side dish.

Enjoy!

Nutrition: calories 241, fat 7, fiber 8, carbs 14, protein 6

Sweet Potato Fries

Preparation time: 10 minutes **Cooking time:** 20 minutes
Servings: 2

Ingredients:

- 2 sweet potatoes, peeled and cut into medium fries
- Salt and black pepper to the taste
- 2 tablespoons olive oil
- ½ teaspoon curry powder
- ¼ teaspoon coriander, ground
- ¼ cup ketchup
- 2 tablespoons mayonnaise
- ½ teaspoon cumin, ground
- A pinch of ginger powder
- A pinch of cinnamon powder

Directions:

1. In your air fryer's basket, mix sweet potato fries with salt, pepper, coriander, curry powder and oil, toss well and cook at 370 degrees F for 20 minutes, flipping them once.

2. Meanwhile, in a bowl, mix ketchup with mayo, cumin, ginger and cinnamon and whisk well.
3. Divide fries on plates, drizzle ketchup mix over them and serve as a side dish.

Enjoy!

Nutrition: calories 200, fat 5, fiber 8, carbs 9, protein 7

Corn with Lime and Cheese

Preparation time: 10 minutes **Cooking time:** 15 minutes

Servings: 2

Ingredients:

- 2 corns on the cob, husks removed
- A drizzle of olive oil
- ½ cup feta cheese, grated
- 2 teaspoons sweet paprika
- Juice from 2 limes

Directions:

1. Rub corn with oil and paprika, place in your air fryer and cook at 400 degrees F for 15 minutes, flipping once.
2. Divide corn on plates, sprinkle cheese on top, drizzle lime juice and serve as a side dish.

Enjoy!

Nutrition: calories 200, fat 5, fiber 2, carbs 6, protein 6

Hasselback Potatoes

Preparation time: 10 minutes **Cooking time:** 20 minutes
Servings: 2

Ingredients:

- 2 potatoes, peeled and thinly sliced almost all the way horizontally
- 2 tablespoons olive oil
- 1 teaspoon garlic, minced
- Salt and black pepper to the taste
- ½ teaspoon oregano, dried
- ½ teaspoon basil, dried
- ½ teaspoon sweet paprika

Directions:

1. In a bowl, mix oil with garlic, salt, pepper, oregano, basil and paprika and whisk really well.
2. Rub potatoes with this mix, place them in your air fryer's basket and fry them at 360 degrees F for 20 minutes.
3. Divide them on plates and serve as a side dish.

Enjoy!

Nutrition: calories 172, fat 6, fiber 6, carbs 9, protein 6

Brussels Sprouts Side Dish

Preparation time: 10 minutes **Cooking time:** 15 minutes

Servings: 4

Ingredients:

- 1 pound Brussels sprouts, trimmed and halved
- Salt and black pepper to the taste
- 6 teaspoons olive oil
- ½ teaspoon thyme, chopped
- ½ cup mayonnaise
- 2 tablespoons roasted garlic, crushed

Directions:

1. In your air fryer, mix Brussels sprouts with salt, pepper and oil, toss well and cook them at 390 degrees F for 15 minutes.
2. Meanwhile, in a bowl, mix thyme with mayo and garlic and whisk well.
3. Divide Brussels sprouts on plates, drizzle garlic sauce all over and serve as a side dish.

Enjoy!

Nutrition: calories 172, fat 6, fiber 8, carbs 12, protein 6

Creamy Air Fried Potato Side Dish

Preparation time: 10 minutes **Cooking time:** 1 hour and 20 minutes **Servings:** 2

Ingredients:

- 1 big potato
- 2 bacon strips, cooked and chopped
- 1 teaspoon olive oil
- 1/3 cup cheddar cheese, shredded
- 1 tablespoon green onions, chopped
- Salt and black pepper to the taste
- 1 tablespoon butter
- 2 tablespoons heavy cream

Directions:

1. Rub potato with oil, season with salt and pepper, place in preheated air fryer and cook at 400 degrees F for 30 minutes.
2. Flip potato, cook for 30 minutes more, transfer to a cutting board, cool it down, slice in half lengthwise and scoop pulp in a bowl.

3. Add bacon, cheese, butter, heavy cream, green onions, salt and pepper, stir well and stuff potato skins with this mix.
4. Return potatoes to your air fryer and cook them at 400 degrees F for 20 minutes.
5. Divide among plates and serve as a side dish.

Enjoy!

Nutrition: calories 172, fat 5, fiber 7, carbs 9, protein 4

85

Green Beans Side Dish

Preparation time: 10 minutes **Cooking time:** 25 minutes
Servings: 4

Ingredients:

- 1 and ½ pounds green beans, trimmed and steamed for 2 minutes
- Salt and black pepper to the taste
- ½ pound shallots, chopped
- ¼ cup almonds, toasted
- 2 tablespoons olive oil

Directions:

1. In your air fryer's basket, mix green beans with salt, pepper, shallots, almonds and oil, toss well and cook at 400 degrees F for 25 minutes.
2. Divide among plates and serve as a side dish.

Enjoy!

Nutrition: calories 152, fat 3, fiber 6, carbs 7, protein 4

Roasted Pumpkin

Preparation time: 10 minutes **Cooking time:** 12 minutes

Servings: 4

Ingredients:

- 1 and ½ pound pumpkin, deseeded, sliced and roughly chopped
- 3 garlic cloves, minced
- 1 tablespoon olive oil
- A pinch of sea salt
- A pinch of brown sugar
- A pinch of nutmeg, ground
- A pinch of cinnamon powder

Directions:

1. In your air fryer's basket, mix pumpkin with garlic, oil, salt, brown sugar, cinnamon and nutmeg, toss well, cover and cook at 370 degrees F for 12 minutes.
2. Divide among plates and serve as a side dish.

Enjoy!

Nutrition: calories 200, fat 5, fiber 4, carbs 7, protein 4

Parmesan Mushrooms

Preparation time: 10 minutes **Cooking time:** 15 minutes

Servings: 3

Ingredients:
- 9 button mushroom caps
- 3 cream cracker slices, crumbled
- 1 egg white
- 2 tablespoons parmesan, grated
- 1 teaspoon Italian seasoning
- A pinch of salt and black pepper
- 1 tablespoon butter, melted

Directions:

1. In a bowl, mix crackers with egg white, parmesan, Italian seasoning, butter, salt and pepper, stir well and stuff mushrooms with this mix.
2. Arrange mushrooms in your air fryer's basket and cook them at 360 degrees F for 15 minutes.
3. Divide among plates and serve as a side dish.

Enjoy!

Nutrition: calories 124, fat 4, fiber 4, carbs 7, protein 3

Garlic Potatoes

Preparation time: 10 minutes **Cooking time:** 20 minutes

Servings: 6

Ingredients:

- 2 tablespoons parsley, chopped
- 5 garlic cloves, minced
- ½ teaspoon basil, dried
- ½ teaspoon oregano, dried
- 3 pounds red potatoes, halved
- 1 teaspoon thyme, dried
- 2 tablespoons olive oil
- Salt and black pepper to the taste
- 2 tablespoons butter
- 1/3 cup parmesan, grated

Directions:

1. In a bowl, mix potato halves with parsley, garlic, basil, oregano, thyme, salt, pepper, oil and butter, toss really well and transfer to your air fryer's basket.
2. Cover and cook at 400 degrees F for 20 minutes, flipping them once.
3. Sprinkle parmesan on top, divide potatoes on plates and serve as a side dish.

Enjoy!

Nutrition: calories 162, fat 5, fiber 5, carbs 7, protein 5

Eggplant Side Dish

Preparation time: 10 minutes **Cooking time:** 10 minutes
Servings: 4

Ingredients:

- 8 baby eggplants, scooped in the center and pulp reserved
- Salt and black pepper to the taste
- A pinch of oregano, dried
- 1 green bell pepper, chopped
- 1 tablespoon tomato paste
- 1 bunch coriander, chopped
- ½ teaspoon garlic powder
- 1 tablespoon olive oil
- 1 yellow onion, chopped
- 1 tomato chopped

Directions:

1. Heat up a pan with the oil over medium heat, add onion, stir and cook for 1 minute.
2. Add salt, pepper, eggplant pulp, oregano, green bell pepper, tomato paste, garlic power, coriander and

tomato, stir, cook for 1-2 minutes more, take off heat and cool down.

3. Stuff eggplants with this mix, place them in your air fryer's basket and cook at 360 degrees F for 8 minutes.

4. Divide eggplants on plates and serve them as a side dish.

Enjoy!

Nutrition: calories 200, fat 3, fiber 7, carbs 12, protein 4

Mushrooms and Sour Cream

Preparation time: 10 minutes **Cooking time:** 10 minutes
Servings: 6

Ingredients:

- 2 bacon strips, chopped
- 1 yellow onion, chopped
- 1 green bell pepper, chopped
- 24 mushrooms, stems removed
- 1 carrot, grated
- ½ cup sour cream
- 1 cup cheddar cheese, grated
- Salt and black pepper to the taste

Directions:

1. Heat up a pan over medium high heat, add bacon, onion, bell pepper and carrot, stir and cook for 1 minute.
2. Add salt, pepper and sour cream, stir cook for 1 minute more, take off heat and cool down.
3. Stuff mushrooms with this mix, sprinkle cheese on top and cook at 360 degrees F for 8 minutes.
4. Divide among plates and serve as a side dish.

Enjoy!

Nutrition: calories 211, fat 4, fiber 7, carbs 8, protein 3

Eggplant Fries

Preparation time: 10 minutes **Cooking time:** 5 minutes
Servings: 4

Ingredients:

- Cooking spray
- 1 eggplant, peeled and cut into medium fries
- 2 tablespoons milk
- 1 egg, whisked
- 2 cups panko bread crumbs
- ½ cup Italian cheese, shredded
- A pinch of salt and black pepper to the taste

Directions:

1. In a bowl, mix egg with milk, salt and pepper and whisk well.
2. In another bowl, mix panko with cheese and stir.
3. Dip eggplant fries in egg mix, then coat in panko mix, place them in your air fryer greased with cooking spray and cook at 400 degrees F for 5 minutes.
4. Divide among plates and serve as a side dish.

Enjoy!

Nutrition: calories 162, fat 5, fiber 5, carbs 7, protein 6

Fried Tomatoes

Preparation time: 10 minutes **Cooking time:** 5 minutes
Servings: 4

Ingredients:

- 2 green tomatoes, sliced
- Salt and black pepper to the taste
- ½ cup flour
- 1 cup buttermilk
- 1 cup panko bread crumbs
- ½ tablespoon Creole seasoning
- Cooking spray

Directions:

1. Season tomato slices with salt and pepper.
2. Put flour in a bowl, buttermilk in another and panko crumbs and Creole seasoning in a third one.
3. Dredge tomato slices in flour, then in buttermilk and panko bread crumbs, place them in your air fryer's basket greased with cooking spray and cook them at 400 degrees F for 5 minutes.
4. Divide among plates and serve as a side dish.

Enjoy!

Nutrition: calories 124, fat 5, fiber 7, carbs 9, protein 4

Cauliflower Cakes

Preparation time: 10 minutes **Cooking time:** 10 minutes
Servings: 6

Ingredients:

- 3 and ½ cups cauliflower rice
- 2 eggs
- ¼ cup white flour
- ½ cup parmesan, grated
- Salt and black pepper to the taste
- Cooking spray

Directions:

1. In a bowl, mix cauliflower rice with salt and pepper, stir and squeeze excess water.
2. Transfer cauliflower to another bowl, add eggs, salt, pepper, flour and parmesan, stir really well and shape your cakes.
3. Grease your air fryer with cooking spray, heat it up at 400 degrees, add cauliflower cakes and cook them for 10 minutes flipping them halfway.
4. Divide cakes on plates and serve as a side dish.

Enjoy!

Nutrition: calories 125, fat 2, fiber 6, carbs 8, protein 3

Creamy Brussels Sprouts

Preparation time: 10 minutes **Cooking time:** 25 minutes
Servings: 8

Ingredients:

- 3 pounds Brussels sprouts, halved
- A drizzle of olive oil
- 1 pound bacon, chopped
- Salt and black pepper to the taste
- 4 tablespoons butter
- 3 shallots, chopped
- 1 cup milk
- 2 cups heavy cream
- ¼ teaspoon nutmeg, ground
- 3 tablespoons prepared horseradish

Directions:

1. Preheated you air fryer at 370 degrees F, add oil, bacon, salt and pepper and Brussels sprouts and toss.
2. Add butter, shallots, heavy cream, milk, nutmeg and horseradish, toss again and cook for 25 minutes.
3. Divide among plates and serve as a side dish.

Enjoy!

Nutrition: calories 214, fat 5, fiber 8, carbs 12, protein 5

Cheddar Biscuits

Preparation time: 10 minutes **Cooking time:** 20 minutes
Servings: 8

Ingredients:

- 2 and 1/3 cup self-rising flour
- ½ cup butter+ 1 tablespoon, melted
- 2 tablespoons sugar
- ½ cup cheddar cheese, grated
- 1 and 1/3 cup buttermilk
- 1 cup flour

Directions:

1. In a bowl, mix self-rising flour with ½ cup butter, sugar, cheddar cheese and buttermilk and stir until you obtain a dough.
2. Spread 1 cup flour on a working surface, roll dough, flatten it, cut 8 circles with a cookie cutter and coat them with flour.
3. Line your air fryer's basket with tin foil, add biscuits, brush them with melted butter and cook them at 380 degrees F for 20 minutes.
4. Divide among plates and serve as a side.

Enjoy!

Nutrition: calories 221, fat 3, fiber 8, carbs 12, protein 4

Zucchini Fries

Preparation time: 10 minutes **Cooking time:** 12 minutes
Servings: 4

Ingredients:

- 1 zucchini, cut into medium sticks
- A drizzle of olive oil
- Salt and black pepper to the taste
- 2 eggs, whisked
- 1 cup bread crumbs
- ½ cup flour

Directions:

1. Put flour in a bowl and mix with salt and pepper and stir.
2. Put breadcrumbs in another bowl.
3. In a third bowl mix eggs with a pinch of salt and pepper.
4. Dredge zucchini fries in flour, then in eggs and in bread crumbs at the end.

5. Grease your air fryer with some olive oil, heat up at 400 degrees F, add zucchini fries and cook them for 12 minutes.
6. Serve them as a side dish.

Enjoy!

Nutrition: calories 172, fat 3, fiber 3, carbs 7, protein 3

Conclusion

Air frying is one of the most popular cooking methods these days and air fryers have become one of the most amazing tools in the kitchen.

Air fryers help you cook healthy and delicious meals in no time! You don't need to be an expert in the kitchen in order to cook special dishes for you and your loved ones!

You just have to own an air fryer and this great air fryer cookbook!

You will soon make the best dishes ever and you will impress everyone around you with your home cooked meals!

Just trust us! Get your hands on an air fryer and on this useful air fryer recipes collection and start your new cooking experience! Have fun!

Lightning Source UK Ltd.
Milton Keynes UK
UKHW020939150822
407319UK00011B/2021